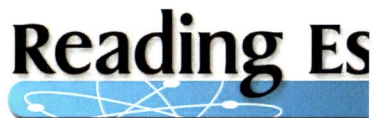

HUMAN BODY BASICS

Bones

CHRISTINE WEBSTER

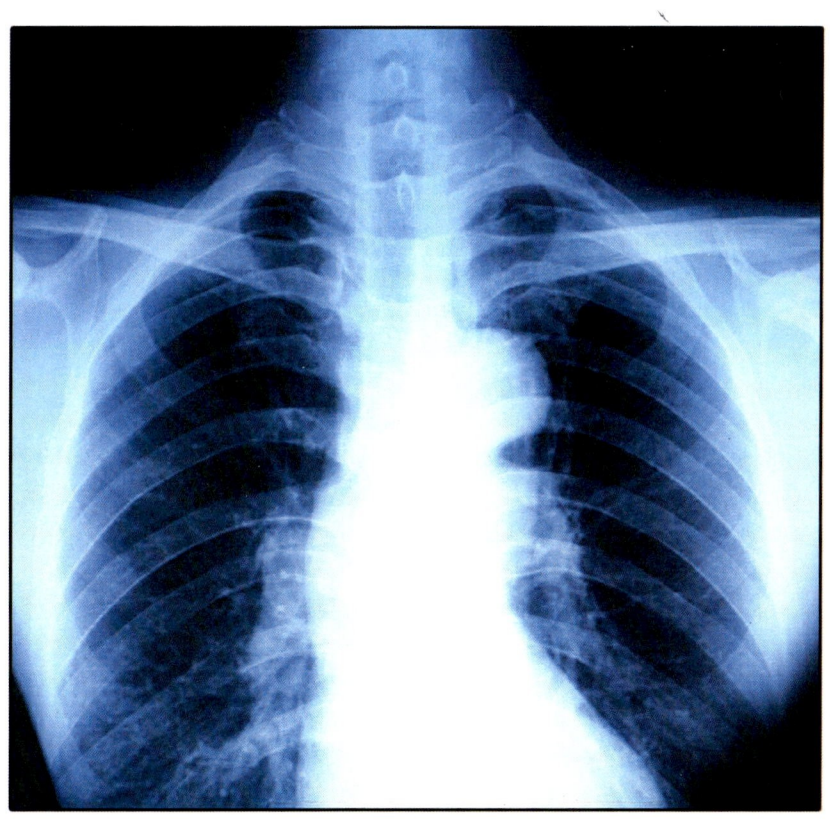

PERFECTION LEARNING®
Children's Home Society

Editorial Director:	Susan C. Thies
Editor:	Mary L. Bush
Design Director:	Randy Messer
Book Designer:	Mark Hagenberg
Cover Designer:	Michael A. Aspengren

A special thanks to the following for his scientific review of the book:
Paul Pistek, Instructor of Biological Sciences, North Iowa Area Community College

Dedication
Thank you, Joan, for your enthusiastic support and constant encouragement.

Image credits
© Bettman/CORBIS: p. 15 (right)

Photos.com: cover (background, left, and right), pp. 3, 4 (top), 6, 7, 11, 12, 13, 16, 17 (top), 22, 24; LifeArt: cover (center), pp. 4 (bottom), 5, 8, 9, 10, 14, 15 (left), 17 (bottom), 18, 19, 20

Text © 2006 by **Perfection Learning® Corporation**.
All rights reserved. No part of this book may be reproduced, stored in a retrieval system, or transmitted in any form or by any means, electronic, mechanical, photocopying, recording, or otherwise, without prior permission of the publisher. Printed in the United States of America.

For information, contact
Perfection Learning® Corporation
1000 North Second Avenue, P.O. Box 500
Logan, Iowa 51546-0500.
Phone: 1-800-831-4190
Fax: 1-800-543-2745
perfectionlearning.com

11 12 13 14 PP 18 17 16 15

Paperback ISBN-10: 0-7891-6628-3
ISBN-13: 978-0-7981-6628-9
Reinforced Library Binding ISBN-10: 0-7569-4688-3
ISBN-13: 978-0-7569-4688-3

Muscles and Tendons

Bones can't move by themselves. They need muscles to help. Muscles are attached to bones by strong cords called *tendons*. One end of a tendon is attached to a muscle. The other end is attached to a bone. When a muscle pulls on a tendon, the tendon moves the bone.

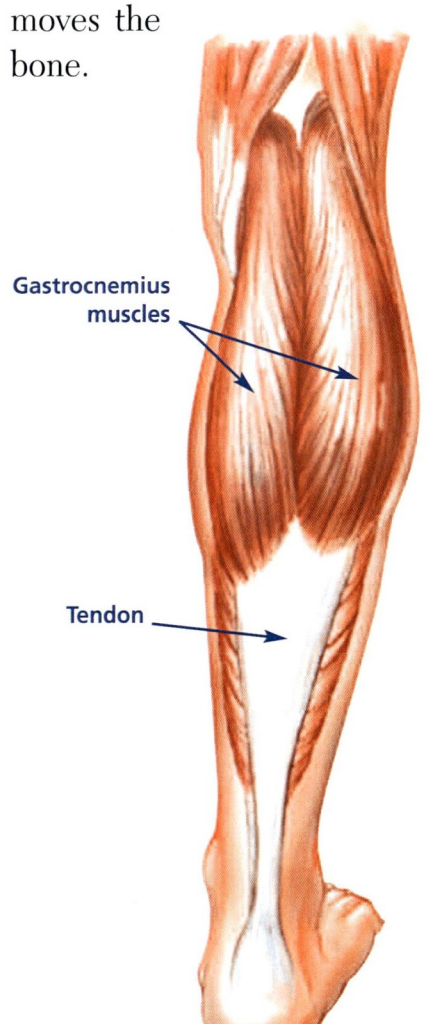

Gastrocnemius muscles

Tendon

Scientist of Significance

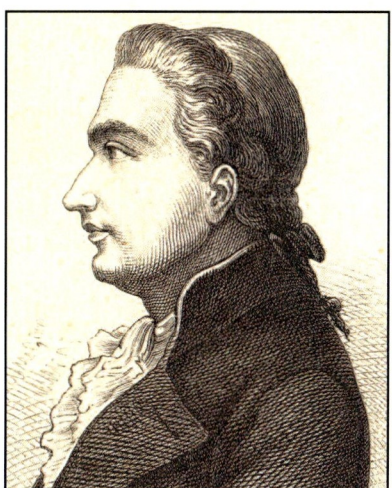

Luigi Galvani made an important discovery in the 18th century. This biologist from Italy used electricity to produce movement in the leg of a dead frog. This made him believe that something electrical causes muscles to move.

Galvani's experiments led to many discoveries by other scientists. Eventually they came to understand that the brain sends electrical messages through the nerves in a body. These messages tell the muscles to tighten or relax. As they do, the bones attached to the muscles move.

Going the Wrong Way

Skeletons are built to withstand normal movement and pressure. But even though bones are strong and flexible, sometimes the wrong movement can cause injury. When twisted, snapped backward, or hit too hard, bones can break.

A broken bone is known as a fracture. A simple fracture is a broken bone that doesn't break through the skin. When the broken bone pokes through the skin, it's a compound fracture. This type of break is more dangerous because germs can enter the body through the opening.

When a bone is broken, a doctor will use X rays to line up the broken pieces. Then a cast, pins, or wires hold the bones together until they heal. New bone growth will repair the edges where the bone broke. In time, the new bone will be as strong as the original.

Technology Link

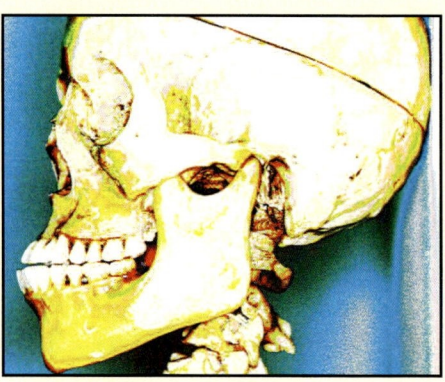

Raymond V. Damadian invented the MRI (magnetic resonance imaging) machine. An MRI takes high-quality pictures of bones and tissue. To have an MRI, a person lies still inside a large, hollow tube. This tube is actually an **electromagnet**. The MRI machine receives signals from the body's tissue. A computer changes these signals into images for doctors to study.

An MRI can scan for broken bones and tears in muscles, tendons, and joints. It is used to scan other body parts, such as the brain and heart, too. Doctors also use MRIs to look for cancer cells in patients.

MRIs are safer and more effective than X rays. However, they take more time and are more expensive.

CHAPTER FIVE

A Bony Body

The 206 bones of the skeleton can be divided into different groups. Each group has a special name and job.

Topping It Off

The skull, or head, is made up of the cranium and the face. The cranium acts as a helmet for the brain. There are normally 28 bones that make up the skull. These bones include those in the middle ear.

The lower jawbone is the only bone in the head that moves. It can open and shut to talk or move side to side to chew.

A Little Bitty Bone

The smallest bone in the body is in the middle ear. It's called the *stirrup*. This tiny bone is only about one-tenth of an inch long.

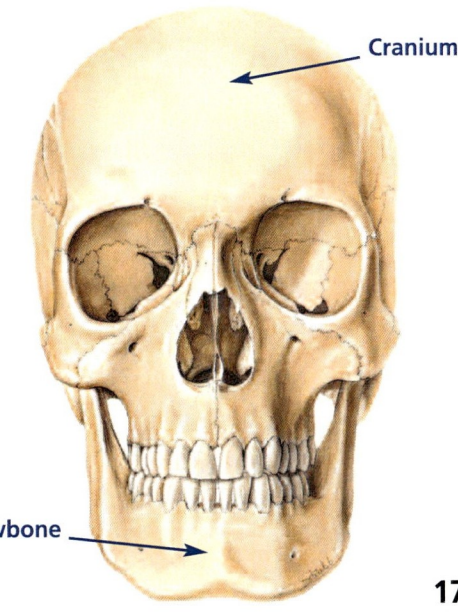

Cranium

Lower jawbone

A Long Way Down

The spine is attached to the head and travels down the back. It is made up of 26 bones called *vertebrae*. In between each of these ring-shaped bones are small disks of cartilage. The cartilage acts as a cushion for the vertebrae.

The spine has several jobs. It holds the body upright and allows bending and twisting motion. It also protects the spinal cord, a bundle of nerves that sends information from the brain to the rest of the body.

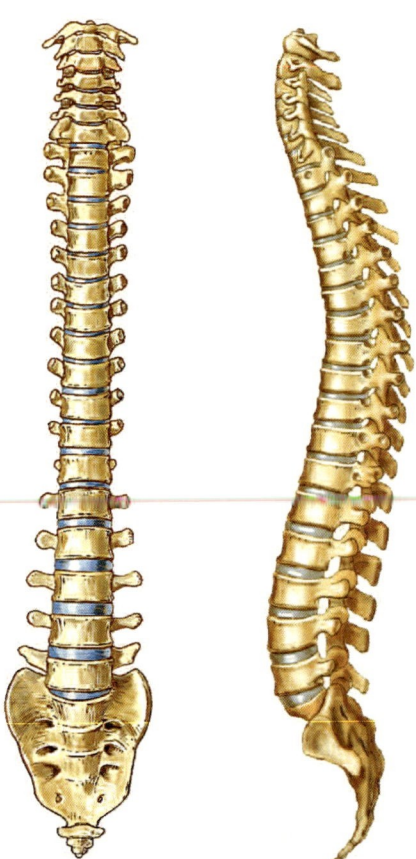

Spine (front view)   Spine (side view)

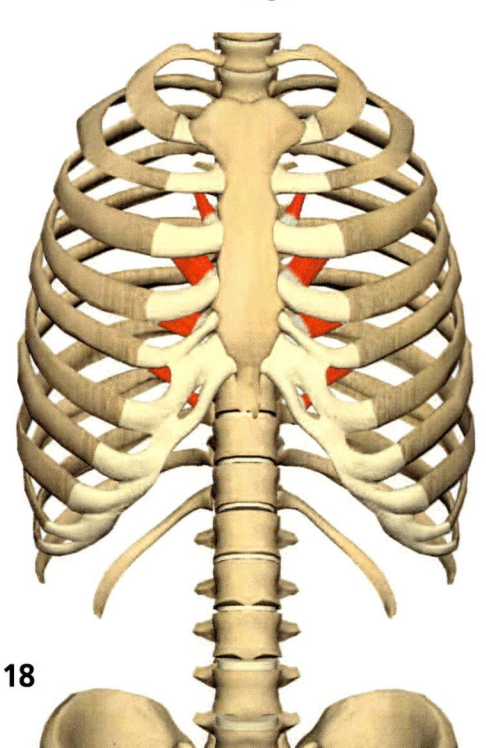

Rib cage

A Safety Cage

Most people have 12 pairs of ribs. These bones form a cage around the heart and lungs. The rib cage protects these important organs from injury. The rib cage expands and relaxes when a person breathes in and out.

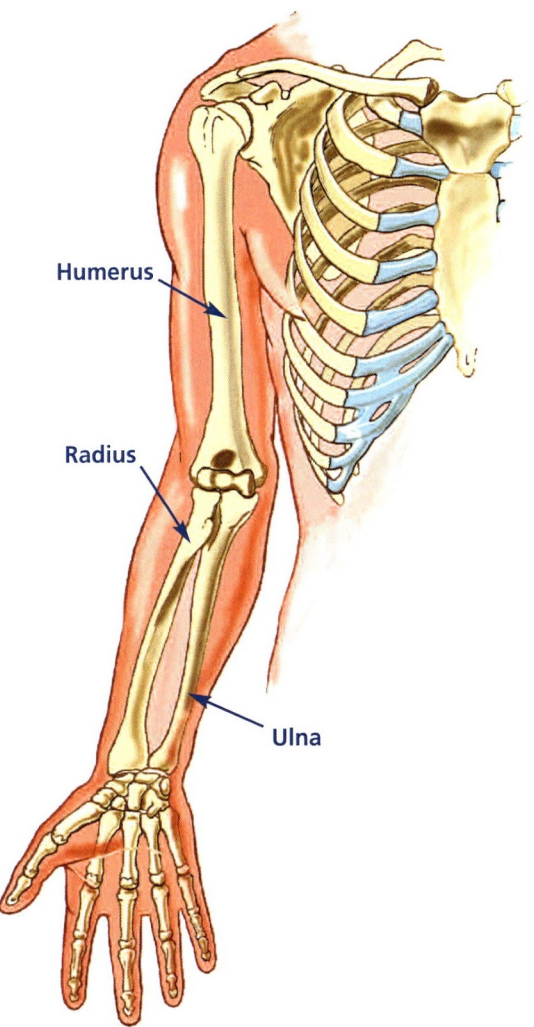

Eight smaller knobby bones make up each wrist. Five separate bones make up the center of each hand. Each finger has three bones. Each thumb has only two bones. All together, there are 54 bones in both wrists and hands. It takes a lot of bones to help you grasp, clench, or throw!

On the Go

The pelvis, legs, and feet are responsible for walking, running, jumping, and dancing. The leg bones are attached to a group of bones called the *pelvis*. The pelvis helps support the spinal column and connects the legs and feet to the rest of the skeleton. The pelvis also protects the bladder, the lower part of the large intestine, and parts of the **reproductive system**.

Leg bones need to be big and strong enough to support the weight of the body. The femur, or thighbone, runs from the pelvis to the knee. It is the longest bone in the body.

Grasp This

The bones in the arms and hands make it possible to lift a bat or throw a ball. The arm is made up of three bones—the humerus, radius, and ulna. The humerus bone is above the elbow. The radius and ulna run side by side below the elbow.

The kneecap is a triangular-shaped bone called the *patella*. The kneecap is part of the joint that connects the femur to the tibia. The fibula is a smaller bone located behind the tibia.

The ankle is similar to the wrist but made up of fewer bones. It has three large bones and four small ones.

Finally, the feet complete the skeleton. Feet may be small, but they have a big job. The bones in the feet balance and support the weight of the entire body.

The bones in the feet are similar to those in the hands. Each foot has five bones. Three bones make up each of the eight smaller toes. Two bones are found in each big toe.

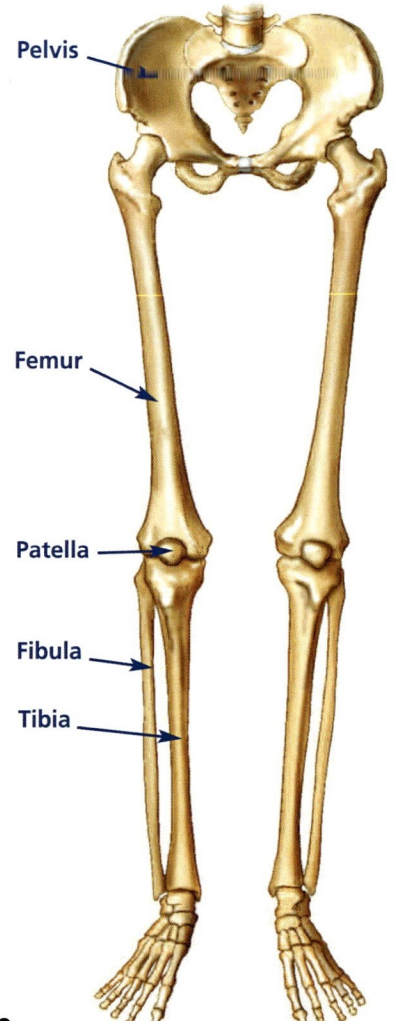

Pelvis
Femur
Patella
Fibula
Tibia

A Finger and Toe Tip

The bones in your fingers and toes are both called *phalanges* (fuh LAN jeez).

From Head to Toe

From head to toe, bones really are incredible. They give you shape, protection, and movement. And all they ask for in return is some calcium, exercise, and care. Give your bones what they need, and they'll give you a lifetime of action!

Internet Connections for Bones

http://kidshealth.org/kid/body/bones_noSW.html
Get the real story on bones—what they're made of, how they grow, and how they work together in the human skeleton.

http://depts.washington.edu/bonebio/
Bone up on your skeleton biology at this student site from the American Society for Bone and Mineral Research.

http://yucky.kids.discovery.com/noflash/body/pg000124.html
Discover some fun and interesting facts about bones.

http://vilenski.org/science/humanbody/hb_html/skeleton.html
Go on a human body adventure to explore bones' structure and function.

http://www.bbc.co.uk/health/kids/bones.shtml
Find out how bones matter to your body with these facts and diagrams.

http://www.EnchantedLearning.com/subjects/anatomy/skeleton/
Check out the diagram of the major bones in the human body along with the facts on the human skeleton. Includes links to skeleton printouts.

Related Reading for Bones

Bones by Stephen Krensky. This book describes how bones perform different functions as part of the human body. Random House, 1999. [RL 2.5 IL K–3] (3253201 PB 3253202 CC)

Muscles and Bones by Andreu Llamas. Explore muscles and bones in this book from the Human Body series. Gareth Stevens, 1998. [RL 7.1 IL 3–7] (5883800 HB)

Skeleton by Steve Parker. An Eyewitness Science book on the skeleton. Dorling Kindersley, 1988. [RL 5.9 IL 5–9] (5867306 HB)

The Skeleton Inside You by Philip Balestrino. This lively, easy-to-read book explains how the bones of the skeleton are joined together, how they grow, how they help make blood, and what happens when they break. HarperCollins, 1989. [RL 2 IL 1–4] (8133201 PB 8133202 CC)

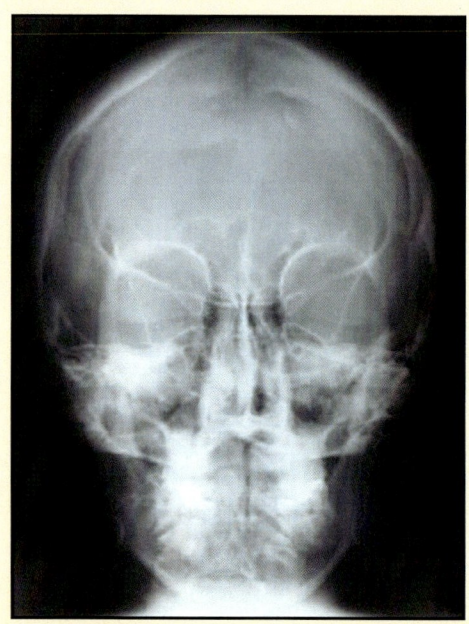

- RL = Reading Level
- IL = Interest Level

Perfection Learning's catalog numbers are included for your ordering convenience. PB indicates paperback. CC indicates Cover Craft. HB indicates hardback.

Glossary

blood vessel (bluhd VES uhl) tube that carries blood around the body

bone (bohn) hard connective tissue that makes up the skeleton (see separate entries for *tissue* and *skeleton*)

cartilage (KAR tuh lidj) tough, flexible tissue (see separate entry for *tissue*)

cell (sel) smallest unit of living matter

crustacean (kruh STAY shuhn) member of a group of animals with jointed legs, a hard outer shell, antennae, and eyes at the end of stalks (lobsters, crabs, crayfish, etc.)

electromagnet (il lek troh MAG net) magnet that gets its attraction from electricity running through it

invertebrate (in VER tuh brayt) animal without a spine (see separate entry for *spine*)

joint (joynt) place where two bones meet

ligament (LIG uh ment) connective tissue that holds bones together (see separate entry for *tissue*)

mineral (MIN er uhl) nonliving substance found in nature

muscle (MUH suhl) body tissue that tenses and relaxes to produce movement (see separate entry for *tissue*)

nerve (nerv) bundle of excitable fibers that connects the brain or spinal cord to other parts of the body

organ (OR guhn) part of the body such as the heart or lungs

platelet (PLAYT let) cell fragment in blood that helps it clot, or stop flowing, when necessary

reproductive system (ree pruh DUK tiv SIS tuhm) team of body parts that works together to create babies

skeleton (SKEL uh tuhn) framework of bones in the body

skull (skuhl) bones of the head, face, and jaw

spine (speyen) series of bones that extend from the head to the bottom of the back

tendon (TEN duhn) connective tissue that attaches muscles to bones (see separate entry for *tissue*)

tissue (TISH you) group of cells of the same kind (see separate entry for *cell*)

Index

Belchier, John, 7
bones
    history, 7
    jobs, 10, 13
    layers, 9
        cancellous bone, 9
        compact bone, 9
        marrow, 9
        periosteum, 9
    number, 5
    shapes, 8
Borelli, Giovanni Alfonso, 7
calcium, 11, 12
cartilage, 5, 18
da Vinci, Leonardo, 7
Damadian, Raymond V., 16
endoskeleton, 6
exercise, 12
exoskeleton, 6
fractures, 16
Galvani, Luigi, 15
joints, 13, 14
ligaments, 13, 14
magnetic resonance
  imaging (MRI), 16
muscles, 13, 15
Roentgen, Wilhelm, 7

skeleton, 4, 17–20
    cranium (skull), 5, 17
    femur (thighbone), 19
    fibula, 20
    humerus, 19
    jawbone, 17
    patella (kneecap), 20
    pelvis, 19
    phalanges, 20
    radius, 19
    rib cage, 18
    stirrup, 17
    tibia, 20
    ulna, 19
    vertebrae (spine), 5, 18
tendons, 13, 15
Vesalius, Andreas, 7

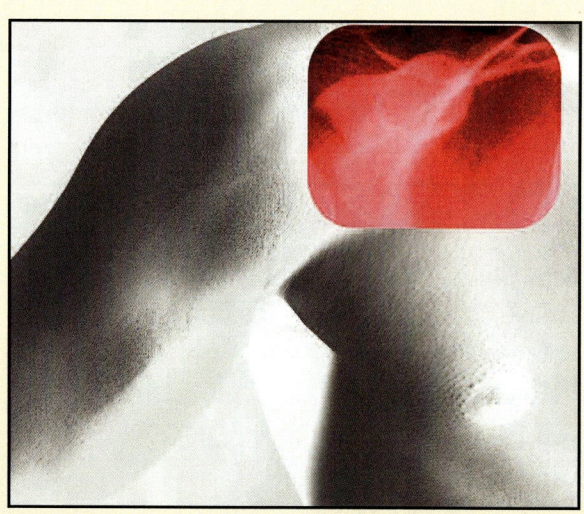

Table of Contents

Chapter One	Born with Bones	4
Chapter Two	Discovering Bones	7
Chapter Three	A Smiling Skeleton	11
Chapter Four	Get Moving!	13
Chapter Five	A Bony Body	17
Internet Connections for Bones		21
Related Reading for Bones		22
Glossary		23
Index		24

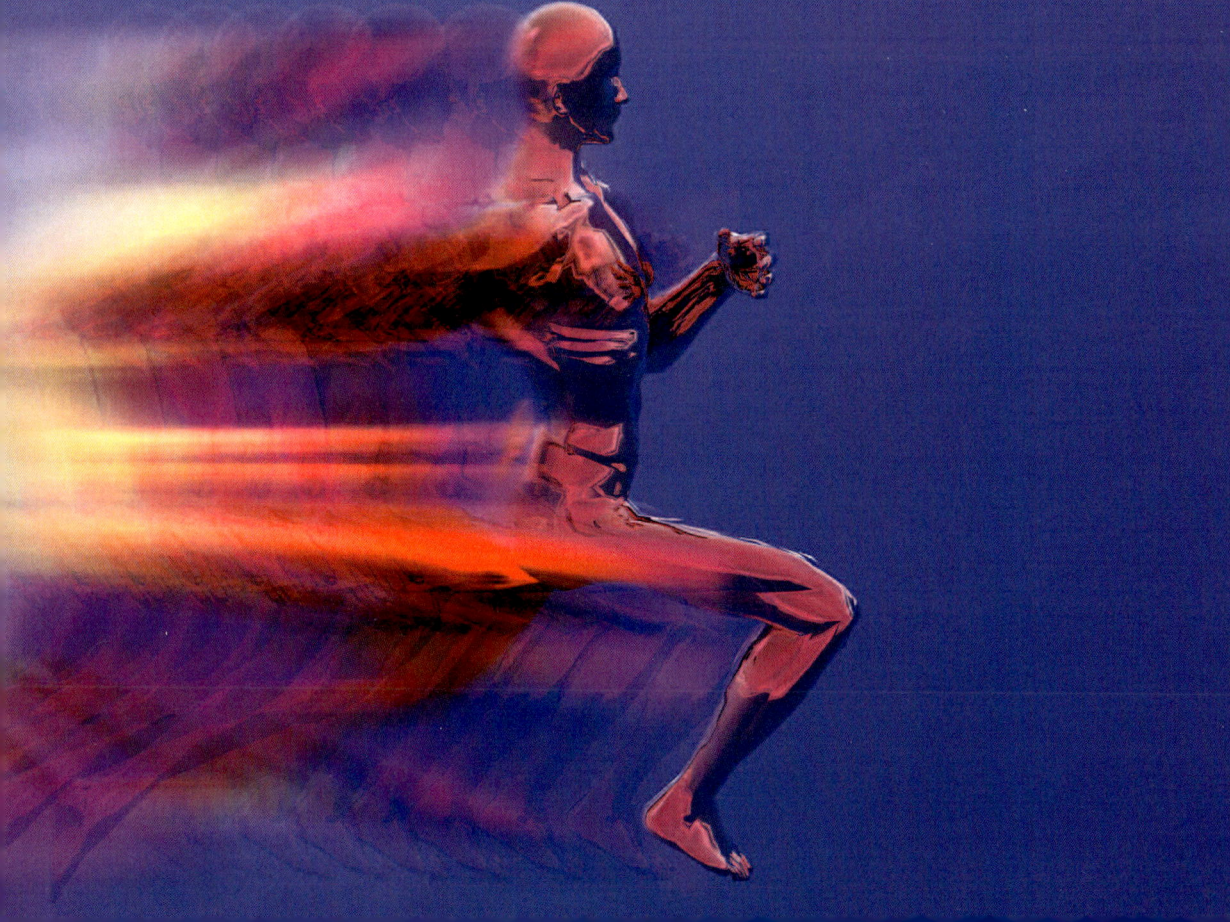

CHAPTER ONE

Born with Bones

Imagine your body without **bones**. What would you become? A heap of skin? A blob of squishy body parts? A river of blood and water? Bones aren't just hard white things that dinosaur scientists dig up or your dog chews. The bones in your body are actually living things with many important jobs. Under your skin, you have an amazing team of bones that works hard to give you shape, movement, and protection.

Hanging Out Together

All of the bones in the body make up the **skeleton**. The skeleton is the framework that holds up and protects all of the other parts of the body.

Before Bones

A baby's bones begin as **cartilage**. This tough, flexible **tissue** eventually changes to hard bone. Many bones complete this change before birth. Others aren't completely hardened until you're in your early twenties.

A few parts of the body are made of cartilage that never changes to bone. The tip of the nose and the outside of the ears are two of these spots.

Disappearing Bones

A baby is born with 300 bones. Most adults have 206 bones. Where do the extra 94 bones go?

As bones grow, many of them fuse, or grow together. For example, a baby's **skull** is made up of 28 separate bones. As a child grows, many of these bones fuse. The same is true in the lower **spine**. Five separate bones in a baby's spine eventually become one.

All of the bones in a human skeleton are completely hardened by age 25. This means that the bones also stop growing. So from this age on, height, shoe size, arm length, and other body measurements stay the same.

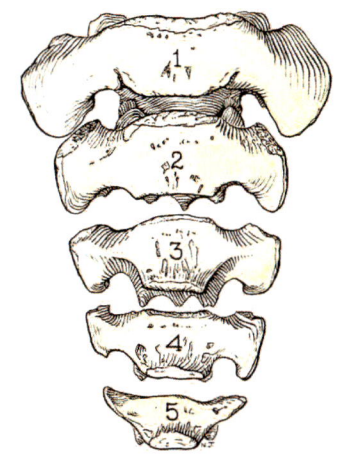

Lower spine of a youth

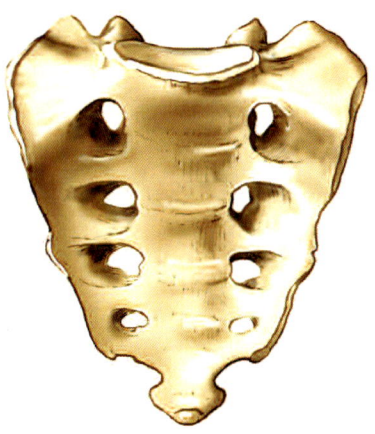

Lower spine of an adult

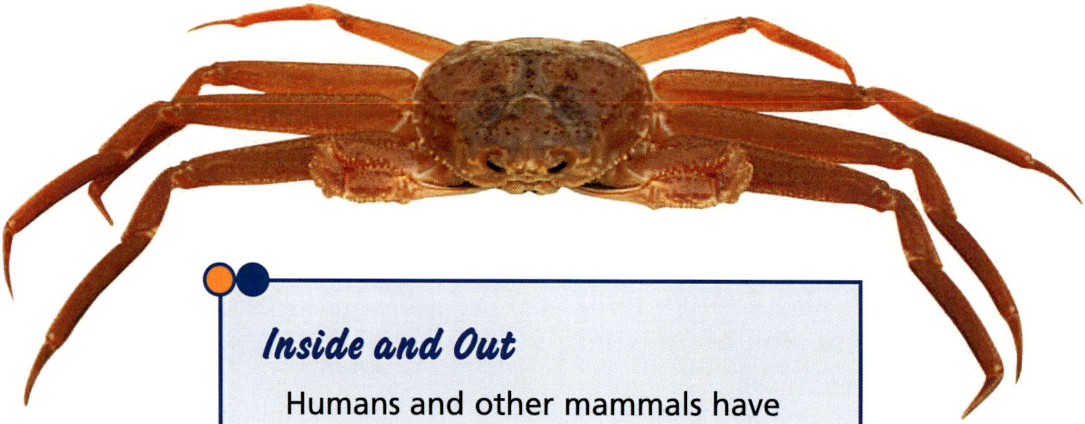

Inside and Out

Humans and other mammals have an endoskeleton. This means that their skeletons are inside their bodies.

Insects, **crustaceans**, and many other **invertebrates** have an exoskeleton. An exoskeleton is found outside the body but does the same jobs as an endoskeleton. For example, a crab has a hard shell on the outside of its body. This skeleton supports the body and protects the crab's insides.

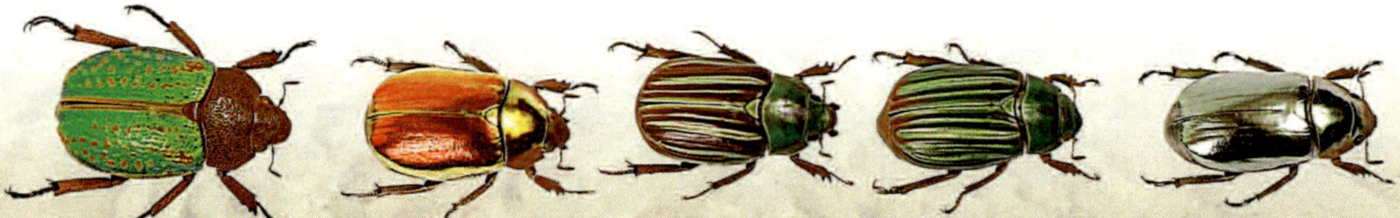

CHAPTER TWO

Discovering Bones

From the beginning of time, people had ideas about bones. They could feel the hard shapes beneath their skin. They saw bones left behind from people and animals that had died. But for a long time, humans didn't truly understand bones. They didn't know what they were made of or what they did for the human body. Over time, advancements in science made these discoveries possible. Today, we have a good understanding of the bones in our bodies.

Skeleton Steps in Time

Late 1400s Leonardo da Vinci drew one of the first drawings of the human skeleton. His pictures showed how bones looked, how they were connected, and how they moved.

1543 Belgian scientist Andreas Vesalius wrote the first book about the human body, including the skeleton.

1670s Giovanni Alfonso Borelli studied how **muscles** move.

1763 An English surgeon named John Belchier measured bone growth.

1895 German physicist Wilhelm Roentgen invented the X ray. This invention enabled scientists to see and study bones in living people.

Shape Up!

Bones come in different shapes and sizes. They can be grouped into four main types—long, flat, short, and irregular. Long bones are shaped like a cylinder, or tube. Leg and arm bones are long bones. Flat bones include the shoulder blades and ribs. Short bones are short and wide. The ankles and wrists have some short bones. Bones with odd shapes are irregular. The bones inside the ear and the bones in the spine are irregular bones.

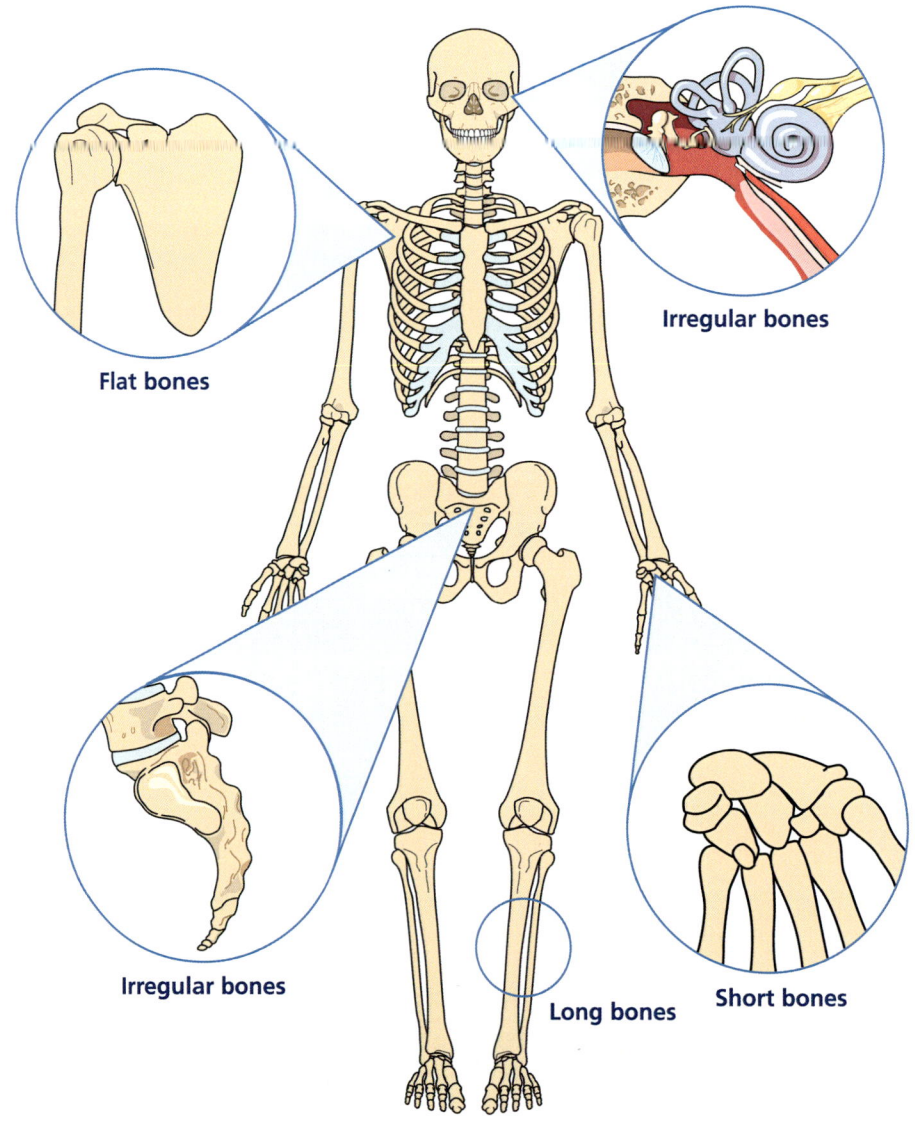

Flat bones

Irregular bones

Irregular bones

Long bones

Short bones

What's Inside?

Bones are living things that grow and change. Bones are made up of water, **minerals**, and living tissue. **Blood vessels** carry food and oxygen to bones to keep them alive and healthy. When a body dies and no longer eats or breathes, the bones die too. So while *your* bones are alive and well, dinosaur bones are not.

Bones are made up of several different layers. A thin protective layer called the *periosteum* covers the outside of a bone. The periosteum is full of **nerves** and blood vessels. This layer protects the bone and helps repair it when injured. It also supplies food and oxygen for the layer beneath it.

Under the periosteum is a white layer called *compact bone*. This part of the bone is very hard.

Underneath the compact bone is spongy bone known as cancellous bone. This layer has many holes in it like a sponge. It is strong but lightweight. This allows bones to support the weight of a body but still move easily.

Spongy bone protects the bone marrow found on the inside of a bone. Bone marrow is a thick, jellylike material that fills in spaces in bones. There are two types of marrow—red and yellow. Red marrow's job is to make blood **cells** and **platelets** for the body. Yellow marrow is mostly fat cells.

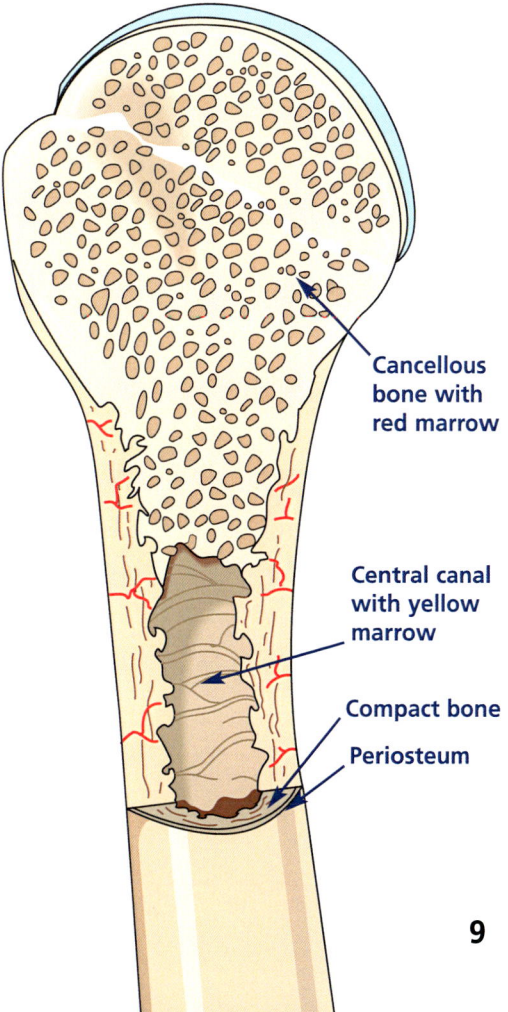

Get to Work!

Bones have several important jobs in the body. Bones support the body and give it shape. They also protect important **organs** like the brain, heart, and lungs.

Bones make and store materials the body needs. The red blood cells made by bone marrow supply your body with oxygen. The white blood cells fight against harmful germs to keep you healthy. The platelets keep you from losing too much blood when you're injured. Minerals, such as calcium and sodium (salt), are stored in the bones until the body needs them.

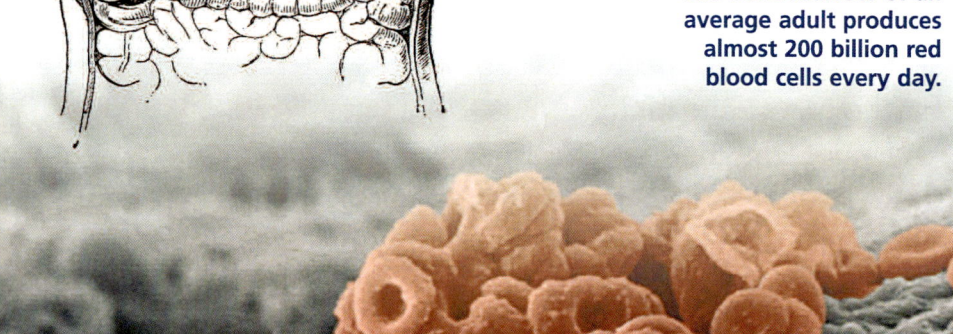

The bone marrow of an average adult produces almost 200 billion red blood cells every day.

CHAPTER THREE
A Smiling Skeleton

Since bones have so many jobs in the body, it's important to keep them strong and healthy. Eating the right foods and getting lots of exercise will help keep your skeleton happy.

Eat Up!

Bones hold almost all of the calcium found in the body. Calcium makes bones strong and helps nerves and muscles do their jobs. It also helps blood clot, or stop flowing, when you cut yourself.

Calcium is found in dairy products. These include milk, cheese, and yogurt. It's also found in leafy green vegetables and eggs.

If you don't get enough calcium, your bones become weak and fragile. They may break more easily and heal more slowly.

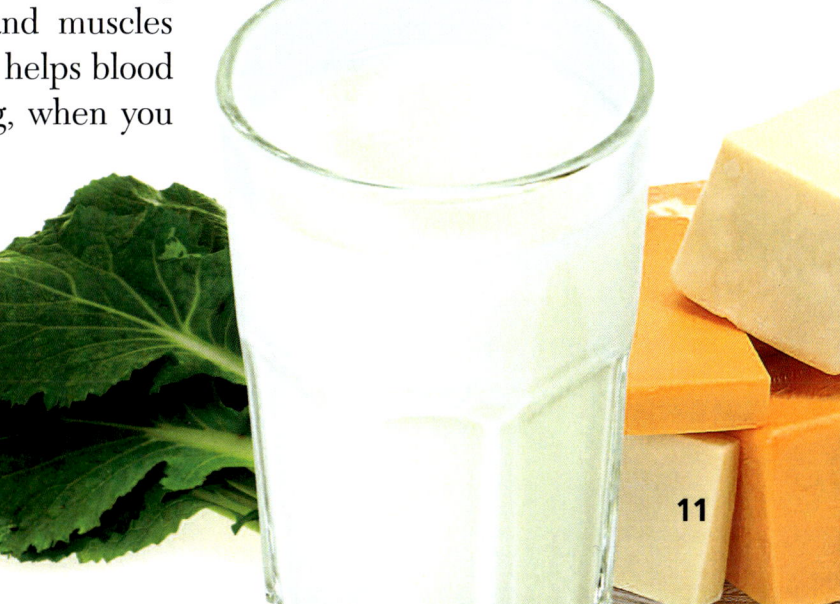

Inquire and Investigate: Calcium in Your Bones

Question: What happens to bones when they lose calcium?

Answer the question: I think that bones _____.

Form a hypothesis: When bones lose calcium, they _____
_____.

Test the hypothesis:

Materials
clean chicken bone
vinegar
small container with a lid

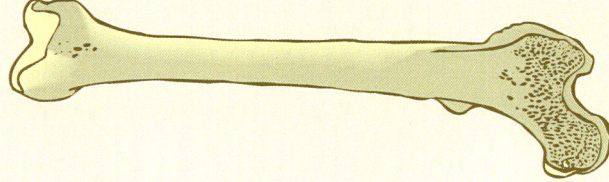

Procedure

Feel and observe the bone. Does it bend? Is it hard or soft? Record your findings.

Place the bone in the container. Cover it with vinegar. The vinegar will remove calcium from the bone.

Close the lid and put the container in a safe spot. Leave it there for two weeks.

After two weeks, remove the bone. Feel and observe the bone now. Does it bend? Is it hard or soft? Compare your findings with those from two weeks ago.

Observations: At first, the bone is hard and doesn't bend. After two weeks in vinegar, the bone is soft, rubbery, and bendable.

Conclusions: When bones lose calcium, they become soft and weak. This is similar to what happens in the body. If you don't get enough calcium in your diet, your body starts taking it from your bones. Eventually, the bones become soft and weak and can break easily.

Exercise Those Bones

You probably know that exercise keeps your heart and lungs healthy. But did you know it also makes your bones stronger and bigger? When muscles pull on bones, the pressure causes the bones to grow thicker and heavier. Athletes who exercise frequently often develop stronger bones than people who sit around watching TV.

CHAPTER FOUR

Get Moving!

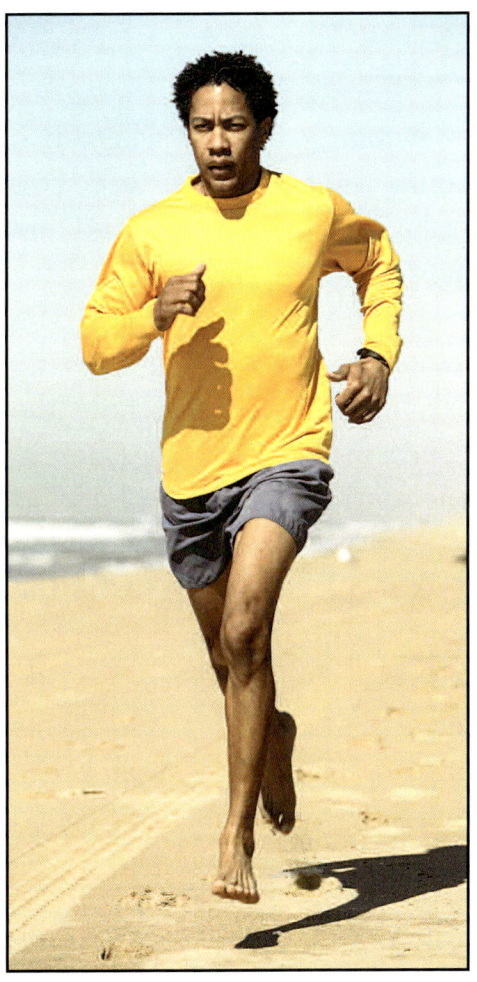

One of the biggest jobs of the skeleton is to give a body movement. To do this, bones team up with other parts in the body.

The Moving Team

If bones were just floating around in your body, they wouldn't be much help when you wanted to move. So what connects bones together and gives them the power to move? These special jobs are done by **joints**, **ligaments**, muscles, and **tendons**.

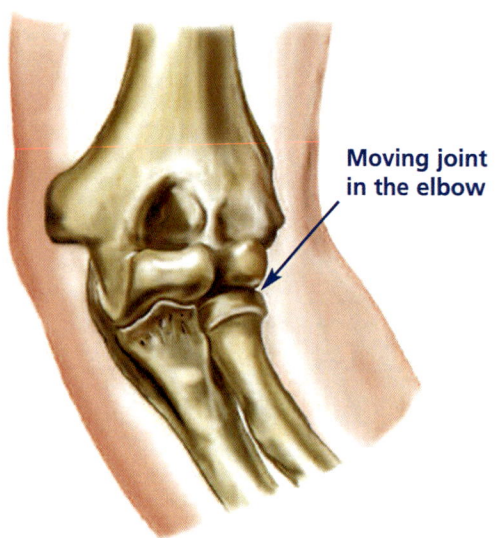

Moving joint in the elbow

Ligaments

Ligaments hold two bones together at a joint. A ligament is a strong, supporting band. Some are long and thin. Others are wide and flat. Ligaments prevent joints from sliding out of place and moving too much.

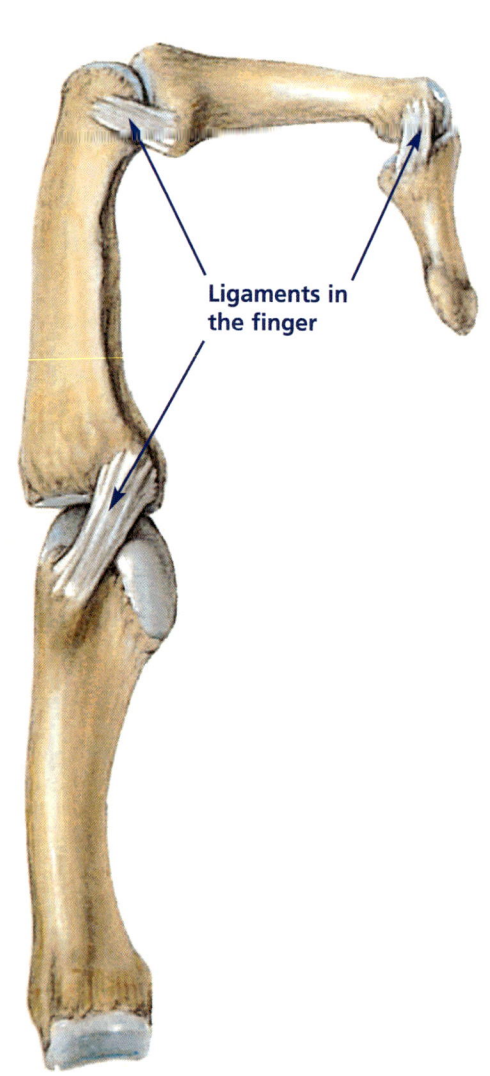

Ligaments in the finger

Joints

A joint is an area where two bones meet. There are two major types of joints—fixed and moving.

Fixed joints don't move. The joints in your skull are an example. These joints hold the bones in the skull together in one solid piece.

Moving joints allow you to walk or play ball or type on the computer. You have moving joints in your arms, legs, neck, hands, and feet. These joints have a special fluid that keeps them moving freely. It's called *synovial fluid*.